YOUR KNOWLEDGE HAS VALUE

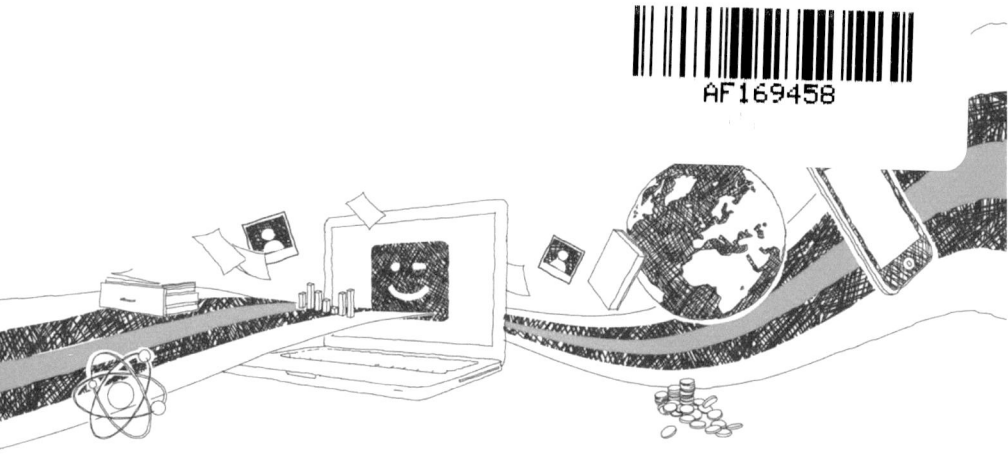

- We will publish your bachelor's and master's thesis, essays and papers

- Your own eBook and book - sold worldwide in all relevant shops

- Earn money with each sale

Upload your text at www.GRIN.com
and publish for free

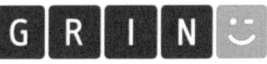

Bibliographic information published by the German National Library:

The German National Library lists this publication in the National Bibliography; detailed bibliographic data are available on the Internet at http://dnb.dnb.de .

This book is copyright material and must not be copied, reproduced, transferred, distributed, leased, licensed or publicly performed or used in any way except as specifically permitted in writing by the publishers, as allowed under the terms and conditions under which it was purchased or as strictly permitted by applicable copyright law. Any unauthorized distribution or use of this text may be a direct infringement of the author s and publisher s rights and those responsible may be liable in law accordingly.

Imprint:

Copyright © 2018 GRIN Verlag
Print and binding: Books on Demand GmbH, Norderstedt Germany
ISBN: 9783668690325

This book at GRIN:

https://www.grin.com/document/421645

Patrick Kimuyu

Impacts of Genetically Modified Food and Alternatives

GRIN Verlag

GRIN - Your knowledge has value

Since its foundation in 1998, GRIN has specialized in publishing academic texts by students, college teachers and other academics as e-book and printed book. The website www.grin.com is an ideal platform for presenting term papers, final papers, scientific essays, dissertations and specialist books.

Visit us on the internet:

http://www.grin.com/

http://www.facebook.com/grincom

http://www.twitter.com/grin_com

Impacts of Genetically Modified Food and Alternatives

Name: Patrick Kimuyu

Table of Contents

Introduction 3
The History of Genetically Modified Seeds 4
The Role of Monsanto in Tackling Global Food Crisis 5
The Problems of Genetically Modified Food 6
    Health Problems Related to Genetically Modified Food 6
    Developmental and Reproductive Toxicity 6
    Allergic Reactions 8
    Antibiotic Resistance 9
Impact on Normal Microflora 9
Environmental Problems 10
    Impact on Ground and Water 10
Alternatives to Genetically Modified Seeds 11
Conclusion 12
References 13

Introduction

In recent years, biotechnology has been the mainstay technology in both agricultural and medical field. This technology has led to the development of new medical techniques such as gene therapy for genetic disorders and diagnostic tools. In the field of agriculture, biotechnology, primarily genetic engineering has led to a substantial breakthrough in food production. It has led to the creation of transgenic plants and animals which express the desired characteristics such as high yield productivity, drought and disease resistance, as well as nutritional profile. In practice, genetic engineered organisms; plants and animals, are created through modifying their wild genomic composition to express new traits (FDA, 2014). These organisms are described as genetically transformed and their genetic composition is relatively different from that of the original or natural organisms referred to as 'wild type.' These genetically engineered plants have been found to enhance food production; thus considered as the modern-day solution to global food crisis. Despite the benefits associated with genetically engineered crops, seeds by Monsanto have been shadowed by immense controversy over safety issues. An endless debate over the safety of genetically engineered seeds has raised an unprecedented outcry over health and environmental concerns. Therefore, this research paper will provide an elaborate discussion on the impacts of genetically modified food.

The History of Genetically Modified Seeds

The history of genetically modified seeds can be folded from 1994 when the first genetically modified crop; the Flavr tomato was approved for commercial purposes by the FDA. However, the events that led to the creation of transgenic seeds have their genesis bears roots from the discovery of recombinant DNA, in 1973. Following the discovery of recombinant DNA, guidelines governing the application of recombinant DNA technology were developed in 1975 during the Asilomar Conference. This led to the issuance of the first GMO patent by the US Patent Office in 1980.

Despite application of recombinant DNA techniques in the medical field, especially the production of insulin from *E. Coli*, this technology appeared in the agricultural field in 1994 when transgenic tomato was introduced in grocery stores. This tomato had been modified to have a long shelve life compared to the conventional tomatoes. However, Monsanto Company was reported to have modified a plant cell in 1982 (Barlett & Steele, 2008).

In 1985, scientists developed a transgenic plant that had the capacity to resist insect pests. Later in 1994, scientists carried out in-vitro fertilization on corn, and this marked beginning of mass commercial production of genetically modified seeds. This started with the introduction of genetically modified tomato in 1994. Advanced research on pesticide resistant toxins led to the development of Bt (*Bacillus thuringiensis*) corn and potato seeds which were approved in the US for commercial use in 1995. This was followed by the development of the so-called Roundup Ready Soybeans in 1996.

Genetically modified seeds production attracted popularity in 1998 when the 'terminator technology' was introduced by Monsanto, in order to commercialize its seeds and maintain its dominance in the agricultural sector as the leading 'seed gene' giant. This move forced farmers to be purchasing GM seeds every season (Anderson, 2014). Since then, genetically modified seeds for crops such as canola, potato, corn, wheat, and cotton have now been developed (FDA, 2014). For instance, Amflora, a genetically modified potato that produces starch for making adhesives and papers was approved by the European Commission in 2010.

The Role of Monsanto in Tackling Global Food Crisis

Monsanto's innovative technologies in producing genetically modified seeds have led to the popularity of genetically modified food products in the global market. The company is said to have achieved technological breakthrough which in food production through development of genetically modified seeds that reduce the cost of food production. In addition, these innovations have been found to promote mass production of food crops. As such, Monsanto's technologies of generating genetically modified seeds remains the only way of solving global food crisis because it holds the capacity to double agricultural output (Louis, 2009). This aspect is reaffirmed by McKie (2011) who reports that genetically modified crops guarantees survival of the global swelling global population in the future.

Moreover, it is perceived that eliminating food shortages in the world will depend on emerging technologies that promote food production and distribution. Therefore, Monsanto is able to solve global food crisis because it has so far produced high yielding genetically modified crops to boost food production. It has also made remarkable advances in weed control through the production of glyphosate-based herbicides (Louis, 2009).

The Problems of Genetically Modified Food

Despite the benefits of genetically modified foods, especially the capacity to improve agricultural output, in order to achieve food sustainability, GMO products have been associated with controversies. From a practical approach, biomedical and environmental safety assessment studies reveal a substantial harm caused by genetically modified foods. Therefore, these foods have been confirmed to cause health and environmental harm.

Health Problems Related to Genetically Modified Food

Currently, genetically modified foods are available in agricultural food supply chains. In the US where genetically modified foods have been approved, genetically modified food products account for over 70 percent, ranging from fresh farm produce to processed industrial food products. Therefore, revelations of health safety concerns arising from the consumption of genetically modified foods create panic within the nation's population, as well as the global population.

Some of the health issues associated with genetically modified foods, which have been identified are antibiotic resistance, allergic reactions, interference with normal microflora, and toxicity.

Developmental and Reproductive Toxicity

According to experimental studies, genetically modified foods have been found to cause reproductive and developmental toxicity in mammals including humans. For instance, experimental investigations involving rats indicate that soy feed causes reproductive problems in female rats. Rats involved in these studies were found to have abnormal heat cycles and gestation problems. This implies that genetically modified soy feed contain some ingredients that interfere with the endocrine system in mammals. Moreover, some rats who were fed with genetically modified soy feed died within 21 days after the initiation of the experiments, implying that the mutated soy feed caused toxicity in the rats. Similarly, newborn rats were found to die within few days after they were introduced to genetically modified soy feed. Therefore, it is apparent that soy feed causes developmental toxicity in mammals, although this phenomenon has not been investigated in humans.

On the other hand, feeding mice with genetically modified feed was found to cause reproductive toxicity. In some studies, mice who were fed on these feeds were identified to produce deformed sperms (Ermakova, 2006). These study results resonate with investigations which were conducted in Australia in which rats were fed on genetically modified corn. In this study, female rats were reported to produce a lower number of litters compared to those fed on conventional corn. In addition, the sizes of the newborn rats were found to be smaller than the ordinary litter size. Similarly, genetically modified corn has also been found to affect pigs and cows. Cows were reported to become infertile after feeding on mutated corn; whereas pigs carried pseudo-pregnancies, as well as becoming sterile. In relation to the results of these experiments which were aimed at determining the impact of genetically modified foods on mammals, it is confirmed that these foods cause developmental and reproductive toxicity (Domingo, 2007).

From an epidemiologic perspective, genetically modified foods seem to have exerted their impacts on the human population where these products constitute the largest percentage of diet. For instance, demographic trends observed within the US women can be interpreted in relation to the impacts of genetically modified foods. According to Paez, et al (2009), women in the US have been observed to give birth to babies with low weight in which the rates have doubled within the last two decades.

Allergic Reactions

Secondly, genetically modified foods have been reported to cause allergies to people after consumption of their products. This phenomenon has been confirmed through research investigations which have found that some genetically modified foods such as corn and soy contain high levels of allergic proteins. According to Finamore et al (2008), experimental studies have shown that these products interfere with immune system responses; thus leading to allergic reactions in animals. For instance, Bt corn was found to cause immune system changes in mice in a study carried out by the Italian Government in 2008 (Finamore et al., 2008).

Similarly, genetically modified corn and soy products have been confirmed to cause allergies. In the US, some asthmatic causes have been linked to allergic reactions triggered by reactive proteins in modified corn and soy. This phenomenon has been proven in the United Kingdom where allergies related to genetic modified soy were found to have increased by 50% since its introduction into the UK consumer market. These incidences of allergic reactions triggered by genetically modified soy imply that soy products that are prepared from the modified soy contain allergic proteins which are responsible for the observed immune system changes. In contrast, conventional soy does not cause any health issues. Therefore, it is imperative that the current change of epidemiological trends of food allergies and asthma can be attributed to the adverse health impacts of genetically modified foods.

As more genetically modified seeds flood the market, it is worth noting that food related allergies and asthmatic cases might surge upwards; thus leading an unprecedented health crisis. However, this phenomenon will cast its severe consequences on populations which rely on genetically modified foods. In contrast, populations that rely on conventional non-GM foods are not likely going to experience such consequences because natural foods are safe for human consumption.

Antibiotic Resistance

Another significant health problem associated with genetically modified foods is antibiotic resistance. Pusztai (2002) observes that antibiotic resistance by pathogenic bacteria has increased significantly since the introduction of genetically modified foods and additives. In practice, new genetically modified seeds are created through the application gene guns, especially *agrobacterium* in which selection of desired genes involves exposure of donor organisms to high doses of antibiotics. Therefore, it is suspected that gene transfer from genetically modified organisms to harmful bacteria has contributed to antibiotic resistance.

Impact on Normal Microflora

The possibility of horizontal gene transfers creates a substantial health risk to humans, as well as other animals. In theory, new genes expressed by genetically modified organisms are expected to be transferred to normal microflora. For instance, the normal microflora that inhabits human gastrointestinal system are likely to be transformed with pesticide-producing genes expressed by Roundup (Donsky, 2014). In addition, consumption of the so-called New Leaf Superior, a pesticidal potato might cause toxicity to humans (Kerns, 2001). This implies that human systems might become genetic transformation sites where lethal toxins can be produced. As a result, new gastrointestinal diseases are expected to emerge as the outcome of the eradication of the normal microflora and production of toxins (Samsel & Seneff, 2014).

Environmental Problems

Genetically modified seeds have been found to compromise environmental safety. This aspect can be confirmed by the hazardous effects of the Agent Orange which was engineered by Monsanto and other companies (Anderson, 2014). Another incidence associated with adverse environmental consequences can be provided by the impact of genetically modified corn monarch butterflies. Friedlander (1999) reports an incidence in the US where investigators from Cornell University discovered the lethal effect of pollen from genetically modified corn. The consequence for this accidental outcome was the drastic reduction of the population of monarch butterflies. Surprisingly, genetically modified corn has been approved for human consumption despite its threat to the ecosystem.

Impact on Ground and Water

It is also reported that genetically modified crops have devastating environmental impact on soils and water systems. For instance, the impacts of the herbicide Roundup that is generated by Monsanto has been found to destroy soil quality. It destroys the soil profile, as well as its nutritional composition (Donsky, 2014). As a result, the ground where this herbicide is grown becomes unproductive because food crops do not flourish leading to reduced agricultural production. In such scenario, the use of genetically modified seeds appears to exert a negative impact on food production.

On the other hand, genetically modified crops have been found to cause water pollution. For instance, pesticide-producing crops scatter pollen into water systems causing contamination. The fact that pollen from genetically modified corn caused toxicity to monarch butterflies implies that pollen from Monsanto's glyphosate-based herbicides release toxins into the environment.

Alternatives to Genetically Modified Seeds

One of the most reliable alternatives to genetically modified seeds is the use of the conventional plant breeding. A study carried out by International Maize and Wheat Improvement Center (CIMMYT) which aimed at creating drought-resistant maize that would be suitable for dry environments proved that conventional breeding was more successful than genetic modification (Woodward, 2014).

The second alternative to genetically modified seeds is the commercialization of ordinary foods such as mushroom and traditional herbs. This implies that the adoption of conventional breeding, a safe technology, can improve agricultural output and avert the looming food crisis.

Conclusion

In a brief conclusion, it is apparent that genetically modified crops exert significant impacts. Foremost, these crops have been found to increase food production. As such, it is believed that the use of genetically modified seeds will solve the problem of global food shortages. This is why Monsanto Company, the leading producer of genetically modified seeds is believed to offer reliable innovations in boosting agricultural output (Barlett & Steele, 2008). However, genetically modified foods have been associated with health and environmental consequences. Some of the health issues include toxicity, antibiotic resistance and allergies; whereas environmental issues are destruction of biodiversity, soil quality and water pollution.

Therefore, there is a need for alternatives to genetically modified seeds.

References

Anderson, L., (2014, March 4). *Why Does Everyone Hate Monsanto?* Retrieved from http://modernfarmer.com/2014/03/monsantos-good-bad-pr-problem/

Barlett, D. J., & Steele, J. B., (2008, May). *Monsanto's Harvest of Fear.* Retrieved from http://www.vanityfair.com/news/2008/05/monsanto200805

Domingo, J., (2007). Toxicity Studies of Genetically Modified Plants: A Review of the Published Literature. *Critical Reviews In Food Science And Nutrition* 47(8): 721-733.

Donsky, A., (2014). *What's So Bad About Gmos? Top Ten Reasons To Avoid Them.* Retrieved from

http://naturallysavvy.com/eat/whats-so-bad-about-gmos-top-ten-reasons-to-avoid-them

Ermakova, I., (2006). Genetically modified soy leads to the decrease of weight and high mortality of rat pups of the first generation: Preliminary studies. *Ecosinform* 1: 4–9.

Finamore, A., et al., (2008). Intestinal and Peripheral Immune Response to MON810 Maize Ingestion in Weaning and Old Mice. *J. Agric. Food Chem.*, 56 (23): 11533–11539.

Friedlander, B., (1999, April 19). Toxic pollen from widely planted, genetically modified corn can kill monarch butterflies, Cornell study shows. *Cornell Chronicle.* Retrieved from http://www.news.cornell.edu/stories/1999/04/toxic-pollen-bt-corn-can-kill-monarch-butterflies

Herbicide on Human Health. Pathways to Modern Diseases. *Global Research.* Retrieved from http://www.globalresearch.ca/monsanto-roundup-the-impacts-of-glyphosate-herbicide-on-human-health-pathways-to-modern-diseases/5342520

Kerns, T., (2001). *Environmentally Induced Illnesses: Ethics, Risk Assessment and Human*

Rights. Jefferson, NC: McFarland.

Louis, S. T., (2009, Nov 19). *The Parable of the Sower —the Debate Over Whether Monsanto is a Corporate Sinner or Saint.* Retrieved from

http://www.economist.com/node/14904184

McKie, R. (2011, January 23). *Genetically Modified Crops Are The Key To Human Survival, Says UK's Chief Scientist [Press Release].* Retrieved from

http://www.guardian.co.uk/environment/2011/jan/23/gm-foods-world-population-crisis

Paez, K., et al., (2009). Rising Out-Of-Pocket Spending For Chronic Conditions: A Ten-Year Trend. *Health Affairs* 28(1): 15-25.

Pusztai, A., (2002). Can Science Give Us the Tools for Recognizing Possible Health Risks for GM Food? *Nutrition and Health* 16: 73–84.

Samsel, A., & Seneff, S., (2014, Janurary 2). Monsanto Roundup: The Impacts of Glyphosate

U.S. FDA. (2014). *Questions & Answers on Food from Genetically Engineered Plants.* Retrieved from

http://www.fda.gov/food/foodscienceresearch/biotechnology/ucm346030.htm

Woodward, L., (2014). *Resisting Drought: Conventional Plant Breeding Outperforms Genetic Engineering.* Retrieved from

http://www.gmeducation.org/feeding-the-world/p217989-resisting-drought:-conventional
-plant-breeding-outperforms-genetic-engineering.html

YOUR KNOWLEDGE HAS VALUE

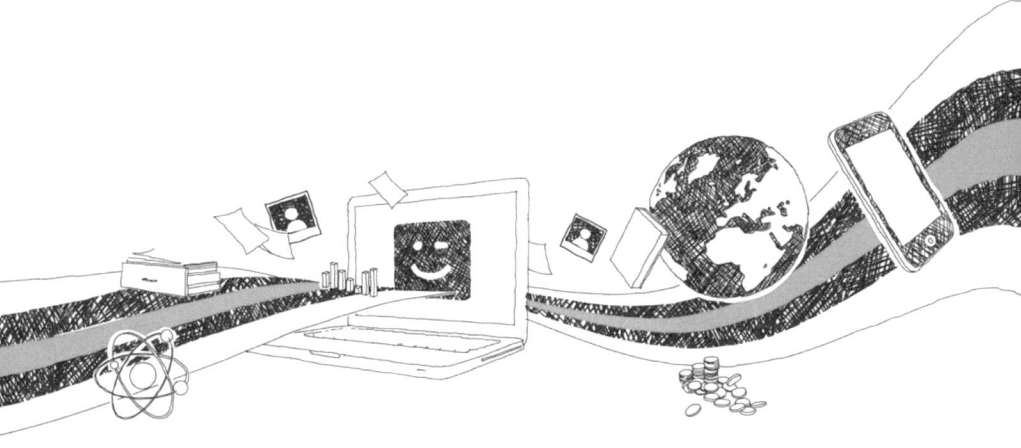

- We will publish your bachelor's and master's thesis, essays and papers

- Your own eBook and book - sold worldwide in all relevant shops

- Earn money with each sale

Upload your text at www.GRIN.com
and publish for free

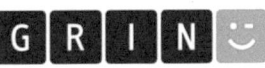